KETOGENIC DIET FOR BEGINNERS

12 SUPER EASY KETO RECIPES

AND A 7 DAY MEAL PLAN

By Rebecca Publishing

Disclaimer

All the material contained in this book is provided for informational and educational purposes only. No responsibility can be taken for any outcomes resulting from the use of this material.

While every attempt has been made to provide information that is both accurate and effective, the author does not assume any responsibility for the accuracy or use/misuse of this information.

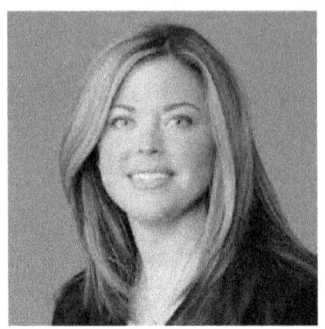

About the author!

I am a newbie to publishing business, but I have a lot of information to tell you. I have been studying healthy way of eating from leading nutritionist in Europe and I have a lot of useful information concerning this topic. I have lost more than 20 kilos so I can provide you with a lot of practical tips on this matter.

My story is also very bright, after giving birth to a child; I gained a lot of extra weight. It was simply impossible to look into the mirror, but I decided to do my best to return myself to my previous shape. I have tried swimming, jogging, different diets like Dukan, Sugar Free Diet, Kremlyovskaya Diet etc. These diets forced me to starving and nothing more. I saw and fell the best result after following the Paleo Diet combined with Ketogenic Diet. This diet helped me to loose ALL my extra weight this is more than 20 kilos/44 pounds and I feel myself much healthier now! I would like to provide you with detailed information about Ketogenic Diet in this book.

Table of Contents

Introduction

Thank you for downloading of my book 31 Proven Steps to Lose Weight plus 23 Healthy Paleo Recipes. If you wish to become slimmer and stay healthy, like people say, to kill two birds with one stone, then this book is the proper thing for you. So let`s begin our way to healthy life with beautiful body?

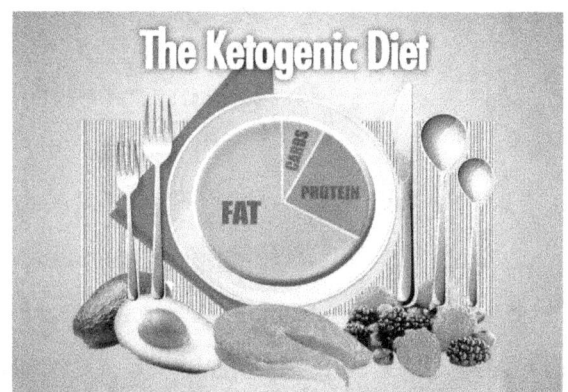

Ketogenic Diet

Eager to be well-turned but not tormented by hunger? Note the Keto Diet! Its unique principles designed just for you! It promises you to break yourself of extra kilos as fast as it possible! Furthermore, you wouldn't suffer from starvation for months. Forget about calories and portions. A Ketogenic Diet is of great mark and mysterious diet for excess weight tired humanity!

Historical information

Keto Diet is not a fashionable novelty. This diet restricts carbohydrates and gives the "green light" fats. First eating plan was evolved by Dr. Russell Wilder at the Mayo Clinic to lend a helping hand children who suffer from epilepsy seizures. It has been clinically tested in the beginning of XX century. During the 1920s-1930s it got popular thanks to its effectiveness, but in the 40-ies - treatment of epileptic attacks by medication became more widespread thus and so the Ketogenic Diet was dead as dodo.

The situation has improved in recent years. The Ketogenic Diet is becoming increasingly popular. What is behind everybody's interest in this diet? People were tired of being fat! This moment humanity was mad about highly powerful method of losing body weight (particularly, losing fat). Quite a number of people have found that this mysterious diet helps them to be rosy about the gills and keep fit. It helped many human beings to work off excess weight, improve health, and to be full of pith.

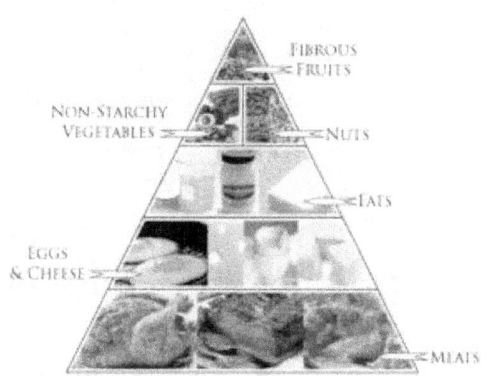

What is a Keto or Ketogenic Diet?

The Ketogenic Diet (or Keto) is a very low-carbohydrate, high-fat diet. Here are ultimate diet tenets

- Eat food which is poor in carbohydrates.

- Eat plenty of fats.

- Have food with a moderate rate of proteins.

Keto-diet bears resemblance to other low-carbohydrate diets. But it is more limited than for example the Atkins diet where you can take any kind of fat. It makes your body to destroy fatty cells (in a form of ketones - bodies, formed as a consequence of fat metabolism) rather than sugar (in a type of glucose/glycogen). This process involves radically reducing carbs consumption, and substituting it with fat. Sharp decrease in carbs brings human organism into a metabolic state which is called ketosis. Usually for these purposes body needs carbohydrates, but in case of their lack, the body finds a solution and resorts to the fats. They are becoming the principal source of energy. Body also transforms fatty cells into ketones in the liver, which can give your brain extra boost.

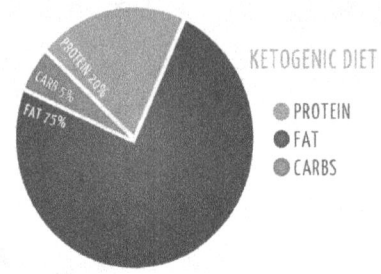

Health Benefits of the Ketogenic Diet

Proven for use that low-cabs diet has a beneficial effect on human health:

•   Heart disease: improves risk coefficients like body fat depositions, tension of blood and blood-sugar levels, HDL levels.

•   Epilepsy: having recurrence to the diet it is possible to lower the percentage of epileptic attacks in kids

•   Cancer: helps to maintain the body of the patients, in a few isolated instances treats varieties of cancer and raises index of tumor growth inhibition.

•   Alzheimer's disease: the diet greatly relieves symptoms of the disease and brakes down progressive illness.

•   Parkinson's disease: as a consequence of taking low-carb, patients suffering from Parkinson's disease feel better

•   Polycystic ovary syndrome: diet menu plan declines insulin levels that is vitally important for patients.

•   Brain injuries: reduces severe concussions of the brain and raises prospect of recovery after cerebral damages.

Choose your Ketogenic Diet!

Pay attention to four varieties of Keto Diet

1)Standard ketogenic diet (SKD): its concept - more fats (around 75%), 20% proteins and 5% carbohydrates.

2)Cyclical ketogenic diet (CKD): alternation of food - five keto-days then two high-carbohydrates.

3)Targeted ketogenic diet (TKD): add carbohydrates around exercise conditioning.

4)High-protein ketogenic diet: duplicate SKD, but requres some more protein. Its tenets - 60% fats, more proteins (around 35%) and 5% carbs.

BUT Only first and fourth kinds of keto-diet are under active consideration. The 2-nd and the 3-d diets - more improved techniques, and mainly musclemen or athletes adhere to its rules.

REMEMBER If you take a Keto-Diet, you shouldn't go beyond the limit of carbs under 30g.

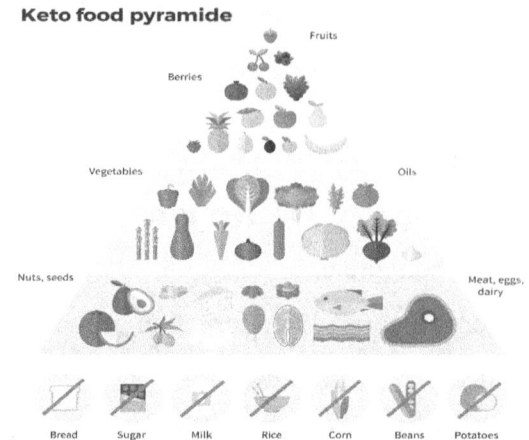

What color of food do you prefer?

Green food - Great: more fats (polyunsaturated or saturated), less carbs.

Blue food - Good: moderate amount of fats, less carbohydrates.

Orange food - Permissible : high fats and moderate quantity of carbs

Red food - Barely permissible: less fats, more carbohydrates.

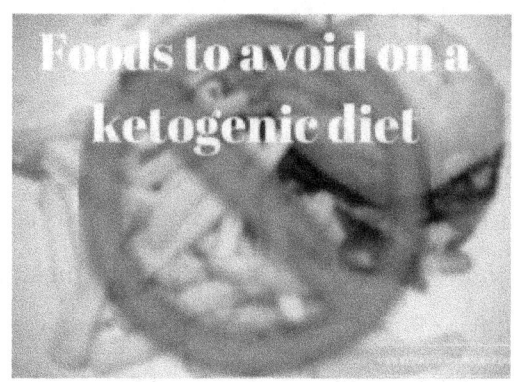

Foods to Avoid

Avoid any factory-farmed meat, food that is rich in carbohydrates, and processed foods.

• Sugary foods: in any form (solid and liquid). This is the main enemy. sugary soft-drinks, candy bars, chocolate, cake, ice cream, candy, fruit juices, table sugar and all items that have extra sugar in them.

• All grains or starches: grain products (loaf bread, any pizza, cookies, buns, crackers), wheat-based food products, barley, rye.

• Dairy products: All the milk-containing product should be avoided. Only a few sips of full-fat, raw milk is allowed. Why milk and dairy products? Milk is poorly digested and it is quite high in carbohydrates (four-five grams of carbohydrates per 100 ml). If you like coffee and tea with milk, replace it with good cream in permissible amounts.

• Fruit: tropical fruits such as pineapples, , bananas, papaya, mangoes etc. and forbidden high-carbohydrate fruits (tangerines, grapes).

• Beans or legumes: lentils, beans, chickpeas, peas, etc.

• Unhealthy fat: refined fats / oils - sunflower oil, soya bean oil, mayonnaise, olive oil, margarine, corn oil.

• Roots and tubers: carrots, potatoes, beat, parsnips, etc.

• Some condiments or sauces: contain sugar and unhealthy fat.

• Alcohol: beer, sweet wine etc. Alcoholic beverages contain a lot of extra calories.

- Low-fat or health food: may be often high in carbohydrates or include gluten, artificial additives, etc

Foods to Eat

Base the majority of your meals around these foods and eat freely:

- Meat: lamb, ham, sausage, beef, turkey, chicken, goat, mutton,
- Seafood, fish: fatty fish (salmon, trout, tuna).
- Eggs: take eggs enriched with Omega 3.
- Butter and cream: use grass-fed when possible.
- Nuts and seeds: almonds, pumpkin seeds, walnuts etc.
- Greengrocery and vegetables: avocados, law-carbohydrate vegetables such as peppers, onions, tomatoes, broccolis.
- Beverages and Condiments: still water, coffee (black or with coconut milk or cream), black or herbal tea, homemade condiments (mayonnaise, mustard, pesto) with no additives, garlic, pepper, high quality sea salt and various safe spices and herbs.

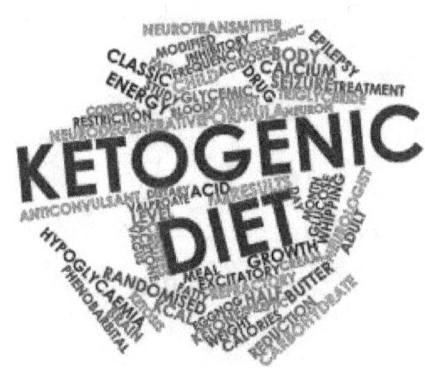

The Ketogenic Diet 7-day menu plan

1st Day – Monday

Breakfast: 2 fried eggs (use coconut oil) and steamed vegetables. One apple or any greengrocery you like.

Lunch: 2 or 3 nuts. Take a chicken salad with an olive oil.

Dinner: Two burgers (if you like) fried in butter and few boiled vegetables or choose salsa.

2nd Day – Tuesday

Breakfast: Have any allowed fruit. 2 eggs with bacon.

Lunch: Two burgers (if you like) that are fried in butter and boil two or more vegetables. Have a fruit mix salad?

Dinner: Fried fatty salmon (use butter). Vegetable mix salad.

3d Day – Wednesday

Breakfast: Chicken, beet, pork or anything meat you like and boiled (steamed) vegetables.

Lunch: Sandwich with a leaf of lettuce; boiled chicken with boiled vegetables.

Dinner: Some berries or nuts, fried beef, grilled vegetables.

4th Day – Thursday

Breakfast: Fried eggs and any low-carbs fruit.

Lunch: Have three or four nuts, a piece of boiled chicken and mixed vegetables.

Dinner: Boiled vegetables and baked meat.

5th Day – Friday

Breakfast: Fried chicken eggs (use coconut oil). and green foods.

Lunch: Some nuts. Chicken salad with an olive oil

Dinner: Take one juicy beef steak with fresh green vegetables and sweet potato for desert.

6th Day – Saturday

Breakfast: Any fresh fruit you like. Eggs with bacon.

Lunch: One beef steak with steamed (or grilled) vegetables.

Dinner: Salmon that is baked in olive oil. One tropic fruit (eg. avocado) and raw vegetables too.

7th Day – Sunday

Breakfast: Boiled carrot, beet etc. and turkey or goat.

Lunch: One sandwich, boiled chicken and fresh raw vegetables salad.

Dinner: Roasted chicken wings (you'd better to use olive oil) combined with boiled vegetables.

Do you believe that you can eat a lot of fatty, delicious and full meal? And at mealtime you lose weight and large volumes? Perhaps this diet is the dream path to the perfect figure!

RECIPES OF DISHES FOR KETO-DIET BREAKFAST (LUNCH)

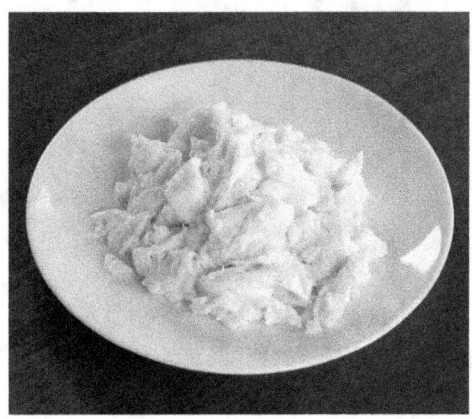

1. Scrambled Eggs

INGREDIENTS

Fresh hen eggs - 3 pcs

Unsalted butter - 1 tblsp.

Salt, pepper

METHOD OF PREPARATION

1. Beat up eggs (better with a fork).

2. Soften the butter.

3. Combine egg mass with butter.

4. Empty out thiis mass into the hot pan.

5. Cook eggs during 60 seconds on one side and then quickly move and cook during one minute on the other side.

6. Scrambled eggs are ready!

7. Put some salt and black pepper!

8. Enjoy hot!

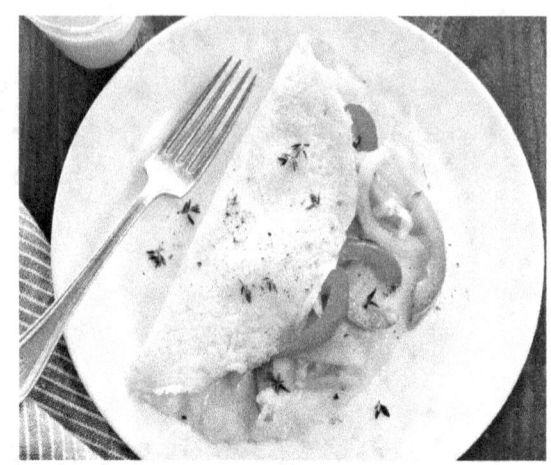

2. Western Omelet

INGREDIENTS:

Hen eggs - 6 pcs

Double cream or heavy sour cream - 2 tblspn.

Salt and pepper

Hard pressed cheese - 130 g

Butter - 56 g

½ yellow onion

½ green bell pepper

Diced ham - 150 g

METHOD OF PREPARATION

1. Blend eggs and cream (sour cream) until they are fluffy. Salt and pepper lightly.

2. Put 75 g of the finally grated hard pressed cheese and mix thoroughly.

3. Let the butter melt in a pan. Then add diced ham, finely chopped onion and pepper. Fry for 1-2 minutes. Add whipped eggs and fry again until ready.

4. Now minimise the temperature and cover the pan. Sprinkle finely grated cheese on top. Turn the omelet on a dish.

5. Serve hot with fresh green lettuce leaves and mild curry!

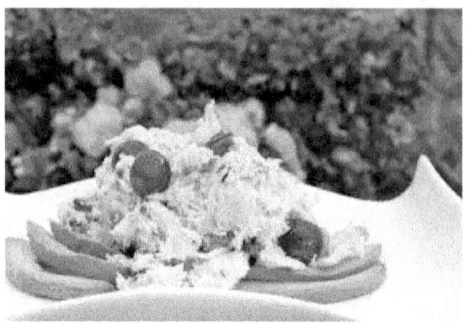

Chicken Salad with Soft Cream

INGREDIENTS:

Diced boiled chicken meat (or duck, turkey) - two glasses

Diced celery - 1/2 glass

Green onion rings - 1/2 glass

Ingredients for Lite Salad Dressing

Liquefied cream cheese - 85 gr.

Dried thyme - 1/2 teaspoon

Mayonnaise (better homemade) - 85 gr.

Dried tarragon - one teaspoon

Freshly ground pepper and salt

METHOD OF PREPARATION

1. Mix liquefied cream cheese and homemade mayonnaise, beat up this mass

2. Put the spices and beat again.

3. Add lite salad dressing to salad components and mix .

4. Add salt (pepper) to taste.

5. Roll up ready salad in green juicy lettuce leaves.

6. Enjoy your eating!

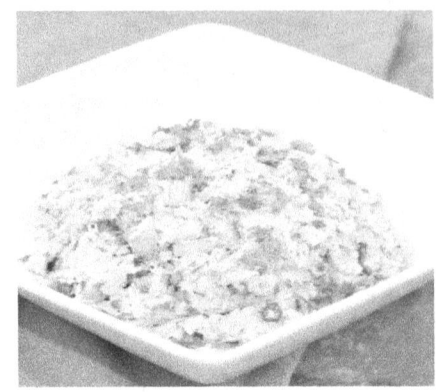

4. Tuna Salad with Capers

INGREDIENTS:

Tuna in olive oil - 1 can

Heavy sour cream - 50 g

Homemade mayonnaise - 180 g

Leeks - 3-5 pcs

Capers (or olives) - 1 tbls

Chili flakes, to taste

Salt and pepper

METHOD OF PREPARATION

1. Drain the oil from canned.

2. Chop leeks.

2. Mix all components: tuna, sour cream, mayonnaise, leeks, capers and flavor with salt, black pepper or chili flakes (or hot chili sauce).

3. Serve with sesame crisp bread and boiled eggs.

NOTE! You may also cut eggs and add directly into the salad. It is tasty to use gherkins, olives instead of capers too.

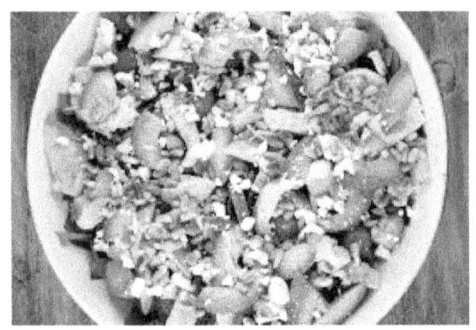

5. Goat-Cheese, Avocado and Bacon Salad

INGREDIENTS:

Goat cheese - 230 g

Bacon- 230 g

Avocados - 2 pcs

Walnuts - 115 g

Arugula lettuce - 115 g

Dressing

Fresh juice of ½ lemon

Homemade mayonnaise - 120 g

Olive oil - 120 g

Double cream - 50 g

METHOD OF PREPARATION

1. Before you start cooking this wonderful salad, switch on the oven and preheat it to 200°C . Place greaseproof paper in a shallow round cake pan.

2. Cut cheese into round slices (about 25 mm) and place in your round cake pan. Bake until golden crust.

3. Take bacon, slice it and fry until crispy.

4. Take an avocado wash it and dry with a paper towel, cut into small blocks.

5. Place arugula lettuce on the plate. On top of the leaves put the   avocado cubs, add the fried crispy bacon and round slices of fried goat cheese. Sprinkle with crushed walnuts.

6. Blend ingredients for a salad flavoring: freshly squeezed lemon juice, 120 g of olive oil, mayonnaise - 120 g and double cream - 50 g. Put a teaspoon of fresh herbs.

7. Salt and pepper to taste.

RECIPES OF DISHES FOR KETO-DIET DINNER (SUPPER)

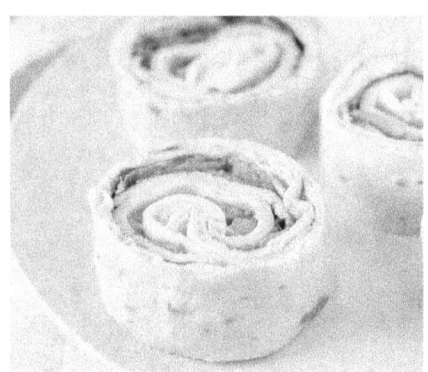

6. Turkey Rolls

INGREDIENTS:

Full-ream cheese - 230 g

Avocado - one piece

Light mayonnaise - one tablespoon

Garlic powder - ¼ tablespoon.

Baked turkey - 450 g

Lemon fresh

Bell pepper - one piece.

Cucumber - two pcs

METHOD OF PREPARATION

1. Soften full-cream cheese at room temperature. Turn it in a deep bowl and lightly beat up until creamy.

2. Carve the avocado in two, remove the pulpy substance. Use the fork and mash it, add one teaspoon of lemon juice. Put salt.

3. Slice cucumber and pepper.

4. Add garlic powder, mayonnaise and the flesh of the avocado to cheese. Mix all this mass for about a minute. Do a thick gravy.

5. Slice turkey meat. Spread meat slices with gravy on both sides, put one or two slices of pepper and cucumber.

6. Make turkey rolls.

7. Cauliflower Casserole in a Delicate Creamy Sauce

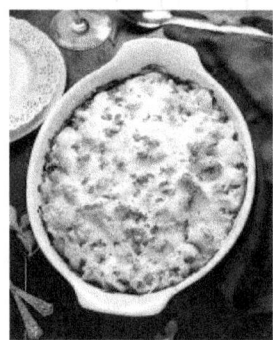

INGREDIENTS:

Fresh cauliflower - 900 g

White onion - 110 g

Butter - 1 tbsp

Cream cheese - 120 g

Heavy cream - 120 ml

Chicken broth - 60 ml

Grated cheese - 100 g

METHOD OF PREPARATION

1. Cut the cauliflower head into small curds. Put them in an enamel pan with lightly salt water and boil cook gently for 20-30 min, until cauliflower become soft and tender. Drain the vegetable and set aside. Or cook the cabbage in a steam cooker.

2. Take a deep pan and put 5 grams of butter. Let it melt. Then add sliced rings of white onion and cook it slowly — until it starts to color.

3.Then add to the fried onion cooked cauliflower. Mixing this mass with spatula, divide curds into smaller pieces. Now minimise the heat and cover the pan.

4. Turn mixture of chicken broth and cream into the pan. Then add cream cheese. Stir slowly ingredients until cheese is melted. You may pour a little more broth if pan's contents get thick. Finally, sprinkle everything with grated cheese. Mix once again.

5.Turn off a fire and shift fried cauliflower together with creamy sauce in a casserole pan, sprinkle finely grated cheese on the top of a dish.

6. Preheat oven to 150 degrees. Bake for 15-20 minutes.

7. Your cauliflower casserole in a delicate cream sauce is ready-to-serve!

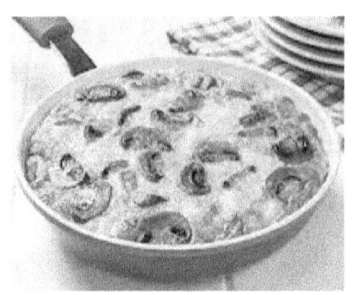

8. Mushroom and Cheese Frittata

INGREDIENTS FOR FRITTATA

Mushrooms - 455 g

Butter - 135 g

Scallions - 6 pcs

Fresh parsley - 1 tblsp

Fine salt - one teaspoon

Ground black pepper - 0,5 tsp

Fresh eggs - 10 pcs

Shredded cheese - 225 g

Mayonnaise - 250 g

Leafy greens - 115 g

INGREDIENTS FOR VINAIGGRETTE SAUCE

Olive oil - four tblsp

White wine vinegar - one tblsp

Salt - 0,5 tsp

Ground black pepper - ¼ teaspoon

METHOD OF PREPARATION

1. Heat up the oven to 175°. Mix together all components for vinaigrette sauce and set aside.

2. Slice, dice or chop the mushrooms.

3. Fry mushrooms in butter until golden (don't forget to mix). Minimise the heat.

4. Finely cut the scallions and combine it with fried mushrooms. Pepper and salt , put one tblsp of fresh green parsley.

5. Blend eggs, grated cheese, mayonnaise in an individual bowl. Put salt and pepper.

6. Grease baking bowl with a butter. Add the mixture of scallions and mushrooms then turn everything into it.

7. Bake about forty minutes or until our delicious frittata gets golden crust and begins pleasantly smell.

8. Cool slightly about 5 minutes and enjoy frittata with leafy green vegetables (eg. spinach)and the vinaigrette sauce.

RECIPES OF KETO-DIET BEVERAGES

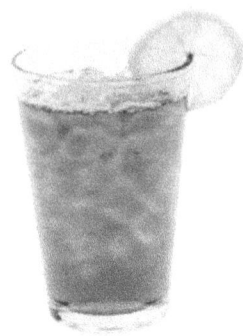

9. Ice Tea

INGREDIENTS:

Cool boiling water - 500 ml

Tea bag - 1 piece

Ice cubes - 1 glass

Slices of lemon, lime

Leaves of fresh mint - 5 pcs

METHOD OF PREPARATION

1. Put 1 tea bag of any type of tea (green, white, yasmin or black), lemon, lime, wedges of orange, tangerine, peach, fresh mint leaves and 250 ml of cool boiling water in a big jug and put in the fridge. Cool about 60-120 minutes.

2. Get the tea bag, wedges of orange, tangerine, peach, slices of lime and green leaves out of the jug. At your wish, you may add variety of fresh flavoring.

3. Pour 250 ml of cool boiling water and serve with lots of cube ice.

4. Enjoy this wonderful tonic drink!

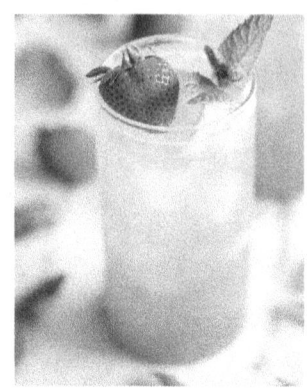

10. Strawberry Lemonade

INGREDIENTS:

Fresh strawberries - 303 g

Lemon juice - 244 g

Substitute for sugar - 200 g

Salt - 1 g

Cold boiling water - 710 g

METHOD OF PREPARATION

1. Take fresh berries, wash them and remove stems. Chop coarsely.

2. Puree the strawberries and other components (except water) in a liquidizer until completely smooth.

3. Turn the fruit puree to a pitcher and dilute with water.

4. Taste and make sweeter as necessary.

5. Mmmm!!! Yummy!!!

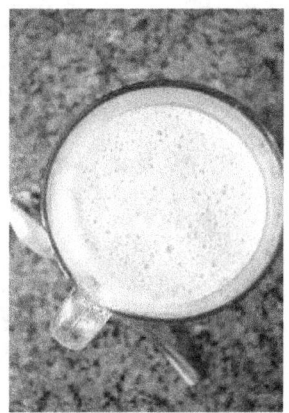

INGREDIENTS:

Fresh eggs - 2 pcs

Coconut oil - 20 g

Boiled water - 12/3 glasses

Vanilla extract - 1 pinch

Ground ginger - 10 g

METHOD OF PREPARATION

1. Blend all components together.

2. Enjoy immediately!

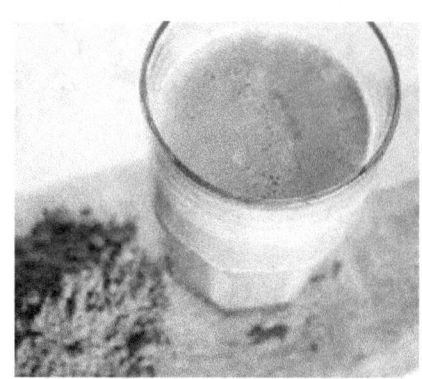

12. Protein Shake

INGREDIENTS:

Whey protein powder

Unsweetened almond milk – 227-453 g

METHOD OF PREPARATION

1. Mix required quantity of whey protein powder and almond milk in the blender bottle
2. If you like add double cream.
3. Ready to drink!

BY THE SAME AUTHOR

You are welcome to read another useful and very informative book by this author!

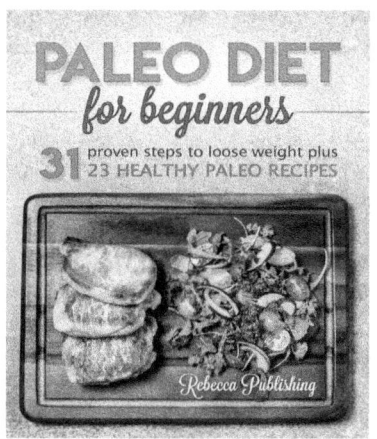

https://www.amazon.com/s/ref=nb_sb_noss?url=search-alias%3Daps&field-keywords=B01MR9UU2O

www.ingramcontent.com/pod-product-compliance
Lightning Source LLC
Chambersburg PA
CBHW081540280526
45788CB00010B/3303